POCKET
EROTIC

DUNCAN BAIRD PUBLISHERS

LONDON

POCKET
EROTIC

THE ECSTATIC SECRETS OF SENSUAL MASSAGE

NICOLE BAILEY

POCKET EROTIC
NICOLE BAILEY

Distributed in the USA and Canada by
Sterling Publishing Co., Inc.
387 Park Avenue South
New York, NY 10016-8810

This edition first published in the UK and USA in 2008 by
Duncan Baird Publishers Ltd
Sixth Floor, Castle House
75–76 Wells Street
London W1T 3QH

Managing Editor: Grace Cheetham
Editor: Dawn Bates
Managing Designer: Manisha Patel
Designer: Saskia Janssen
Commissioned Photography: John Davis

Library of Congress Cataloging-in-
Publication Data available

ISBN: 978-1-84483-707-6

10 9 8 7 6 5 4 3 2 1

Typeset in Futura
Color reproduction by
Colourscan, Singapore
Printed in Hong Kong by Regent

For information about custom
editions, special sales, premium
and corporate purchases, please
contact Sterling Special Sales
Department at 800-805-5489 or
specialsales@sterlingpub.com.

PUBLISHERS' NOTE:
The publishers, the author, and the
photographer cannot accept any
responsibility for any injuries or
damages incurred as a result of
following the advice in this book,
or of using any of the techniques
described or mentioned herein.
If you suffer from any health
problems or special conditions, it is
recommended that you consult your
doctor before following any practice
suggested in this book. Some of the
advice in this book involves the use
of massage oil. However, do not
use massage oil if you are using a
condom—the oil damages latex.

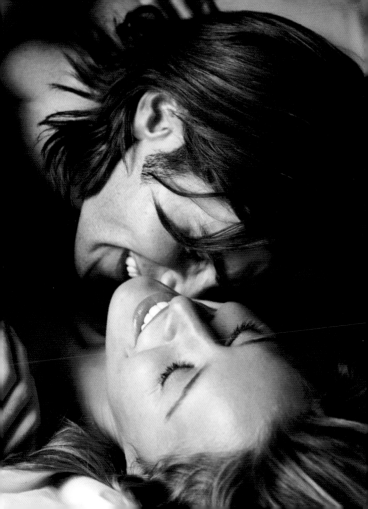

contents

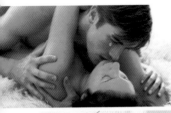

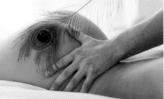

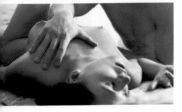

introduction

It is all too easy to forget how to really touch each other. Erotic massage is wonderful – it can bring passion and playfulness, as well as a new connection, eroticism and sensuality to your lovemaking.

At the start of a relationship, it can be hard to keep your hands off each other and you will spend hours in bed discovering what makes each other tick sexually. But when the relationship settles down, it's easy to get out of the habit of touching in ways that truly connect you with each other, and to make assumptions about how your lover wants to be touched.

anyone can do it!

To deliver erotic pleasure through massage, you don't need to attend classes or learn complicated strokes and techniques – you just need to tune in to the sensual power that lies in your palms and fingertips. In fact, it doesn't even have to be in your hands — you can deliver a sublime massage using only your lips, your tongue, your hair, or even your toes. A massage can take all day or it can be as quick and simple as stroking your lover's face and neck before you both go to sleep.

How to use this book

This is a book to look at and read with your lover — let the erotic photography inspire you and take it in turns to choose a particular massage or exercise. If sensual touch has slipped down the list of priorities in your relationship, dedicate one night per week to erotic touch. Light some candles, undress each other, and then open this book at random to see where it takes you! If you've recently met your lover, use the suggestions in this book to enhance your discovery of each other. This book has been divided into three parts – each giving you a slightly different erotic experience. Either work your way gradually through the book, or dip in to your favourite section depending on how the mood takes you.

from hot to red hot

In part 1 – Hot – there is a gradual introduction to sensual touch and erotic massage to help you and your lover discover what you each like and open the lines of sexual communication.

In part 2 – Hotter – the temperature rises as you and your lover delve deeper and look for those truly erogenous zones, as well as learning to get "hot" all by yourself through self-touch. Although the hands are the most obvious massage tool, you'll discover how to use other parts of your body to pleasure your partner.

In part 3 – Red Hot – be prepared to get really down and dirty as you and your lover become more experimental with sex toys and learn some tricks of the tongue that will have your partner begging for these massages every time.

new pleasures

At the end of each section, you'll learn how to use sensual touch while experimenting with a range of different positions, including some from Eastern texts such as the *Kama Sutra* and *Ananga Ranga*.

With the confidence to communicate with each other about how you like to be touched, I hope you will enjoy a renewed openness in your lovemaking and that the erotic touch techniques you'll learn will take you and your lover to new heights of sexual pleasure. Enjoy getting hot together!

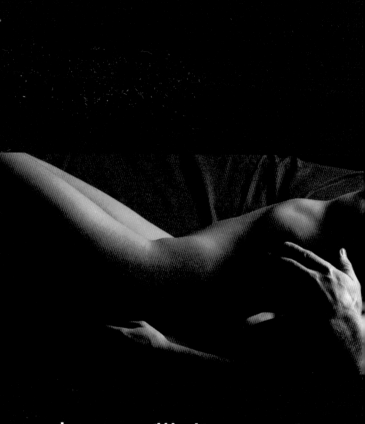

explore • caress • nibble • kiss • tease • excite

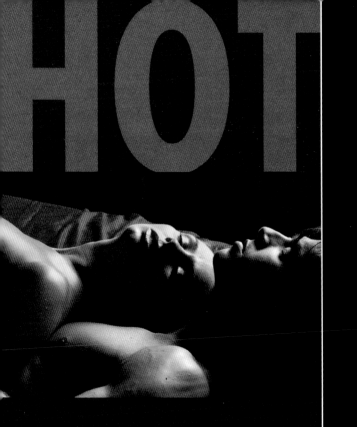

HOT

HOT

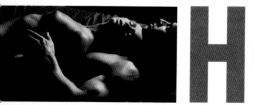

HOT

Heat things up in the bedroom and discover one of

the greatest sensual pleasures in life by exploring

your lover's body through touch. Discover how, by

caressing your lover before and during lovemaking,

you can turn sex from a purely genital experience

into a whole-body experience.

Use the massage techniques in this chapter

to slow down your foreplay, enjoy sensual skin-to-skin

contact, and take time to get to know your lover's body

intimately. Learn how they like to be touched and caressed, pinpoint *all* their hot spots and discover what really turns them on. And find out how giving a sensual massage can be just as pleasurable as receiving one.

Take your lover to new heights of sexual pleasure by experimenting with different touch techniques during lovemaking. Simply hit your lover's erogenous zone at the right time and you will turn good sex into toe-tingling, out-of-this-world sex.

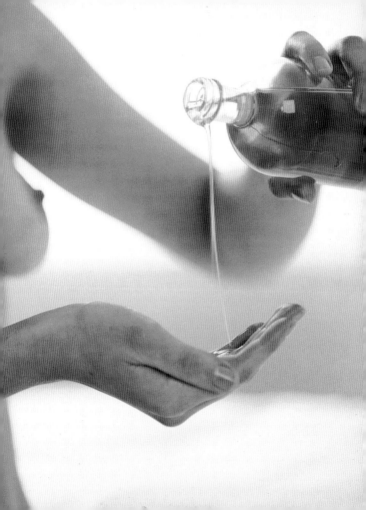

For things to really hot up for you and your lover, they need to start out warm and comfortable. Being in the right environment in which to seduce your lover is everything when it comes to sensual touch. Create a calming, intimate atmosphere by lighting candles, burning incense or essential oils, and playing soft music. Use warm, fluffy towels and make sure your hands are warm too.

warm oil ups

Oil is an important ingredient in a sensual massage — it can stimulate the senses, create an overall more erotic experience for both of you, and make it easier to apply the techniques. Warm the oil before you apply it: rub it between your hands or, if you are using a bottle of oil, let it rest in a bowl of hot water first.

start gently

Massage techniques create a range of wonderful sensations that are both relaxing and stimulating. Start with a more tender touch before moving on to firmer techniques *(see page 20)*.

tender techniques

To use the gliding technique *(see right)*, lay your hands flat and move them smoothly across your lover's skin. This stroke is a good way of letting your hands travel from one part of the body to another.

Now "tap" by curling your hands into loose fists and, using the side or the flat part of the middle of your fingers (not your knuckles), tap your lover's legs, shoulders or back.

Then try the raking stroke: "rake" your fingertips across the skin. This creates a wealth of sensations: fast and hard is arousing and energizing; soft and slow is delicious and sensual.

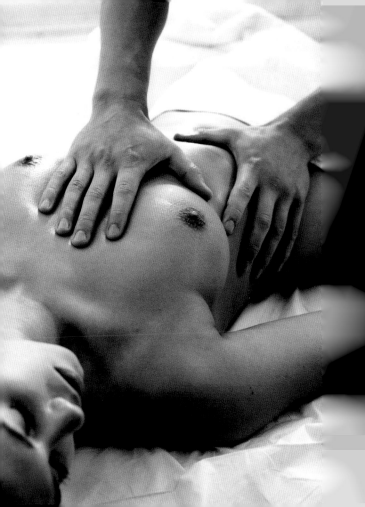

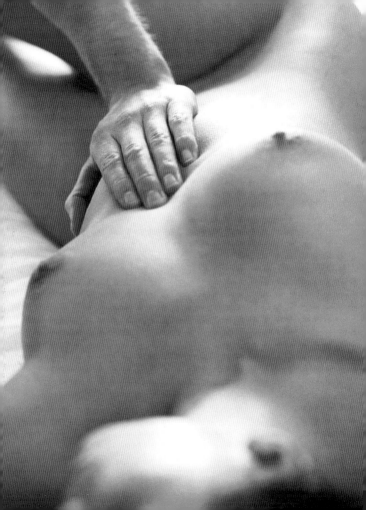

get firmer

Once your lover is relaxed, you can increase the pressure with some deeper techniques. Always ask for feedback and adapt the stroke if necessary. Never put pressure directly on the spine.

deep techniques

Apply pressure gradually by leaning your body weight forward into your hand and pressing firmly with your fingertips *(see left)*. Pressure can be static or circular. As one hand lifts off, your other hand should begin the next stroke to stay in contact with the skin.

Then choose a fleshy part of your lover's body and squeeze it between your fingers and thumbs. Finally, make your hands into fists, rest your knuckles on your lover's body and roll them from side to side, applying pressure as you go. This feels great and effectively relieves muscle tension.

give pleasure

You can master all the massage strokes in the world, but your lover won't enjoy receiving them if they sense you are not enjoying the experience. Giving a massage should be a pleasure and not a chore.

enjoying the experience

If you are feeling tense or uncomfortable, you'll transmit your tension to your lover. Check that your posture is not twisted and that you are not leaning over your lover at a difficult angle. If you are on the floor, kneel on a towel. If your arms or hands begin to ache, use a less penetrating massage stroke for a while.

You won't give a good massage if your thoughts are elsewhere. Tune into your lover and simply think about the pleasure you are giving. If this is difficult, concentrate on your breathing, or try to imagine that you are the person receiving the pleasure.

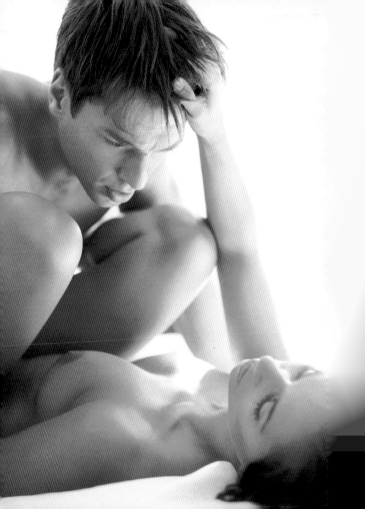

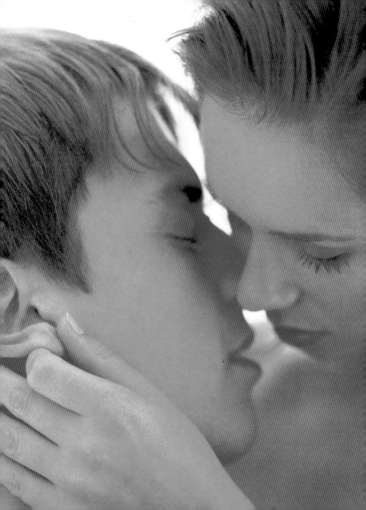

receive pleasure

To get something out of being massaged, you need to put something in. Give yourself up to the experience and make it clear how you want to be touched, and you'll enjoy a great range of sensations.

stilling your mind

A common way to sabotage the pleasure of a massage is to be preoccupied with thoughts or worries, or by thinking about the massage itself. For example, you might be worried that your lover is looking at your body in a critical way.

Bring your attention to your breath. As you inhale, imagine you are taking your breath directly to the area being massaged. Imagine your breath caressing the inside of your body in the same way that your lover is caressing the outside. As you exhale, imagine tension and thoughts floating out of your body.

i want you to

and caress me

explore me...

everywhere

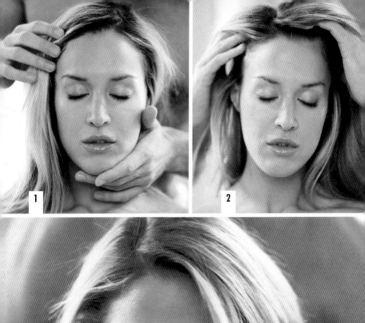

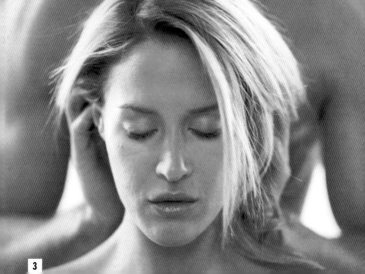

SENSUAL HEAD MASSAGE

A head massage is a sensual and soothing form of massage. It's a great way to nurture each other and create a mood of relaxed, loving intimacy.

1 Ask your lover to sit in a straight-backed chair and close their eyes. Gently place your hands on their shoulders. Take three deep breaths in synchrony with each other. Then gently caress your lover's face with your fingertips – on their forehead, chin and along the cheekbones.

2 Coat your hands in oil and rake your fingers through your lover's hair using long, smooth strokes. Apply light pressure with your fingertips throughout. Repeat this step for several minutes to relax your lover fully.

3 Place your fingertips above your lover's ears and apply gentle pressure in slow circles. Repeat this stroke on your lover's temples. If you prefer, you can use the heels of your hands.

SENSUAL FOOT MASSAGE

The foot is a major erogenous zone for many people. Indulge your lover with this exquisite massage by giving undivided attention to their feet.

1 Rest your fingertips on the top of your lover's foot and position your thumbs on the sole. Now press in tiny circular movements. Do this in the same place for about a minute and then repeat along the length of the foot.

2 Hold the heel of your lover's foot in one hand and, using the thumb of your other hand, press firmly all the way along the underside of the foot. Do this several times.

3 Finish by rotating each foot in circular movements, clockwise and anti-clockwise, around their ankle. Then press their foot firmly between your hands. When you have finished the massage, gently enclose your lover's foot in a warm towel. Then massage the other foot in the same way.

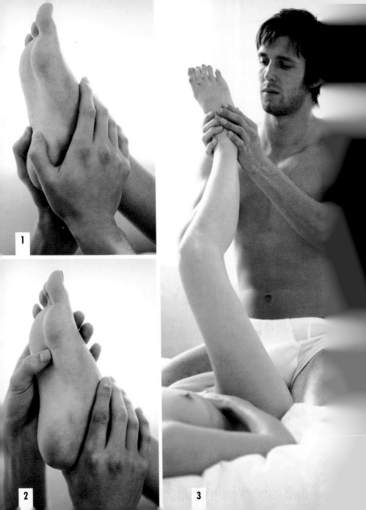

suck me, nibble me

The mouth is a great sensual touch tool so massage your lover by sucking and nibbling. The expectation of pain can cause a frisson of arousal in some, but do make your nibbles playful, not painful.

tantalizing techniques

Show your lover how you like to receive oral sex by giving them "fellatio" or "cunnilingus" on their finger. By watching and feeling what you do, your lover will quickly understand what you want.

Thoroughly lubricate your lover's skin with saliva or oil and then go to bite them. But instead, let your teeth glide across the skin. Softly pinch their flesh and then gently caress it with your teeth. Nibble and graze rather than nip or bite. Create an airtight seal between your lips and your lover's skin then suck and gently graze the skin — beware, this is famous for leaving a tell-tale mark!

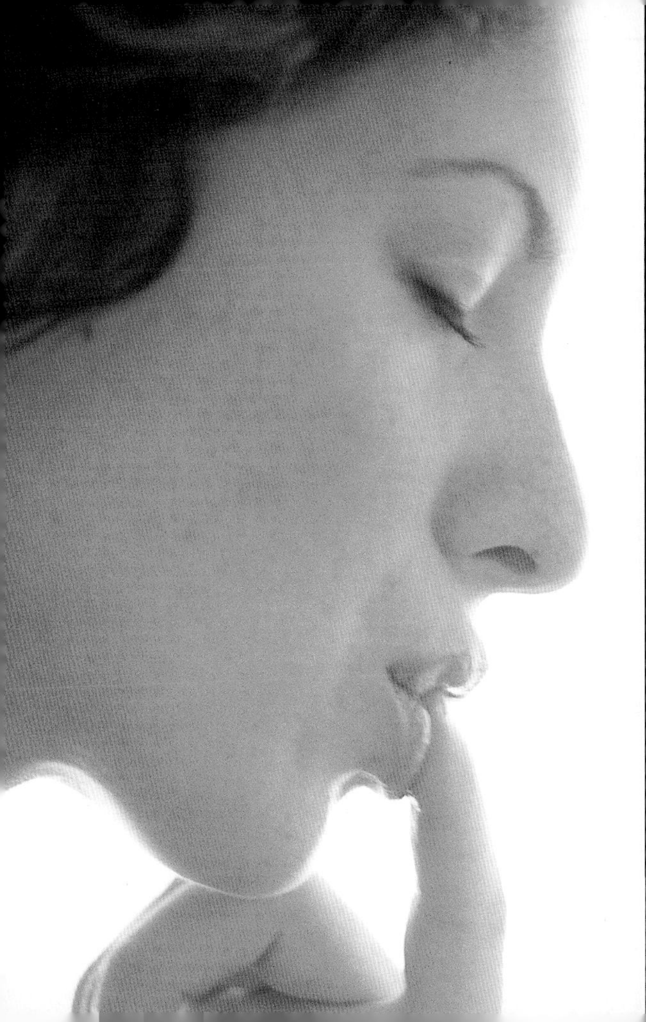

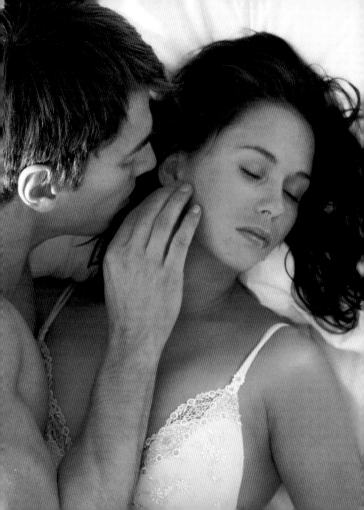

touch me there

You can never know too much about what turns your lover on, and discovering what makes them shiver and tingle is part of this. Tell or show each other how and where you want to be caressed.

hot spots

Create a top five or a top ten list of your favourite hot spots for your lover. Be as honest as you can: while you might find a head, back or foot massage relaxing, it's often more unconventional zones that really turn people on. These might be on your earlobe, behind your knees, in your armpits, along the line of your collar bone, on your wrists, or on your fingertips.

If there are parts of your body where you don't like to be touched, tell your lover about these too as it is important that they are aware of and sensitive about these places.

please tell me

and make it

a fantasy...

really hot

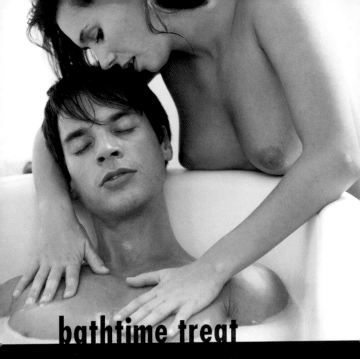

bathtime treat

Take your lover by the hand and lead them to a hot, fragrant, candlelit bath. Instruct them not to speak but just to enjoy the sensual experience of being bathed. Carefully undress your lover and invite them to climb into the bath. Get in too if there's room; otherwise just kneel beside the bath. Cover

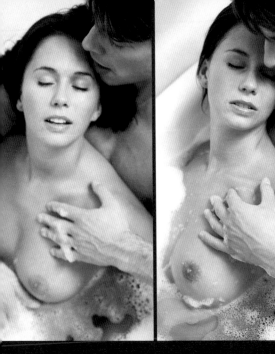

your lover in soapsuds and slowly and sensually wash every part of their body, except for their genitals. Finally, wash this area using lots of gel as a lubricant and fingertip strokes. Invite your lover to step out of the bath. Wrap them in a warm towel and gently dry them. Now remove their towel.

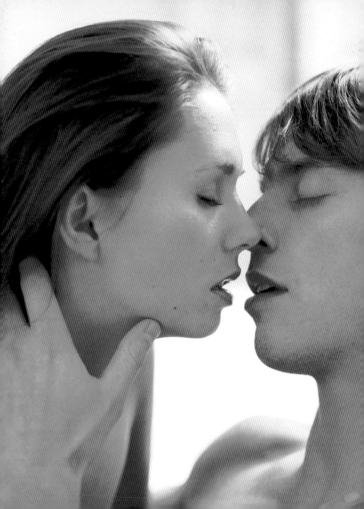

loving breath

Using your breath alone is one of the subtlest and most sensual massage tools imaginable, creating a feeling that is simply sublime and an incredible feeling of intimacy.

Blow Your Lover Away

Face-to-face, feel each other's breath before you kiss. Then ask your lover to lie on their front and gently blow across their buttocks in the direction of their head. Now move so that you are sitting a little higher up their body, take another deep breath and blow out again in the direction of your lover's head. Do this all the way up the spine.

Ask your lover to lie on their back. Now blow the energy back down their body: from the head, across the chest and belly and down to the genitals. Try licking the surface of your lover's skin and then blowing very softly on the moist skin.

AN ENERGY MASSAGE

The aim of this massage is to stimulate your lover's body so they feel tranquil, yet energized. It is a great way to unwind and connect with each other.

1 Ask your lover to lie on their front. Kneel beside them and hold your palms a short distance from the base of their spine. Close your eyes and visualize the energy emanating from their body.

2 Next move your hands in circles above the point at the base of their spine. Then gradually move your hands in circular movements up your lover's spine (still not touching the skin).

3 Move your hands back down to the base of the spine. Now make contact with your lover's skin by resting both hands on the spot at the base of the spine. Circle your hands on this spot. Without taking your hands off your lover's body, slide them up their back and circle them again. Now ask your lover to turn over and repeat the circling motion on the front of their body.

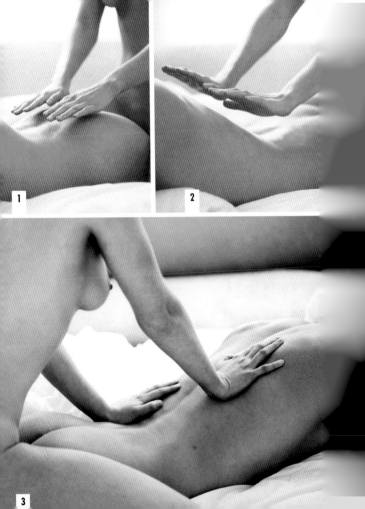

1

2

3

Now that you've both thought about how you want to give and receive massage, try putting it into practice with this sensual awakening exercise.

Explore your lover's body slowly through touch. Begin by tracing the outline of your lover's face with your fingertips. Then try walking your fingers up their thighs, and rolling their fingers between your thumb and forefinger. Experiment with different speeds and pressures. During this stage of the programme, avoid touching your lover's breasts or genitals. That happens at the next stage.

Repeat stage 1, but this time include your lover's breasts and genitals. Your aim is not to bring your lover to orgasm, but to give them a sensual experience that encompasses their whole body. Touch their genitals and breasts in a playful, exploratory way rather than in a way that is familiar, and don't give these areas more attention than the rest of the body.

STAGE 3 Take it in turns to massage each other. As in the previous stages, rather than trying to reach orgasm you're aiming to awaken a new level of sensitivity in each other's body and give each other delicious sensations. Use as much oil as you want, and experiment with props – a silk scarf, a piece of velvet, a soft paintbrush. You don't have to do anything complicated with these objects. Simply sitting behind your lover and brushing their hair in long, smooth strokes, or wafting a silk scarf over their naked skin can be a sensational experience.

STAGE 4 Now you can touch each other at the same time, using oil and props and including the breasts and genitals. This mutual touching takes sensuality and eroticism to the next level because you can both feed off each other's responses. As tempting as it might be to have sex or stimulate each other to orgasm, try to resist. After doing this exercise, describe what you enjoyed and the sensations you felt. Try to maintain and use what you've learned from each stage before and during lovemaking.

do it harder

your role is to fully pleasure your lover, but it won't hurt to listen and familiarize them so they tell you what they really want you to do. Ask them for feedback throughout. This might be in a nonverbal 'mmmm' or single words such as 'nice', 'more' or 'harder' — they should be begging for you to give them more pleasure. If your lover doesn't

give me more

deeper...

pleasure

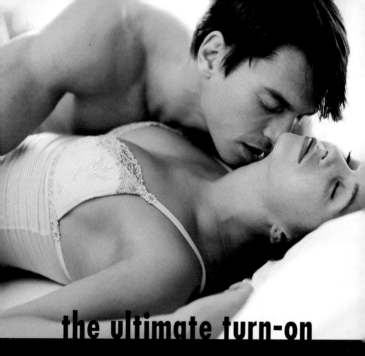

the ultimate turn-on

Tease and tantalize with this combination of kisses and caresses that will take your lover's arousal levels sky-high. Bring your lips close to their ear and gently kiss their temple and the area around the ear. Make your kisses featherlight and barely audible. Gently suck and nibble the earlobe. To

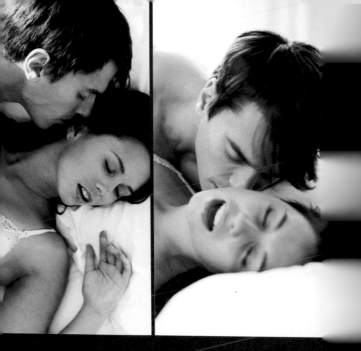

take the eroticism a notch higher, simultaneously caress your lover's nipple. Next, try probing the inside of the ear with the tip of your tongue. Finally, plant a row of exquisitely featherlight kisses from the ear, working your way slowly and sensually down the neck. Now explore further.

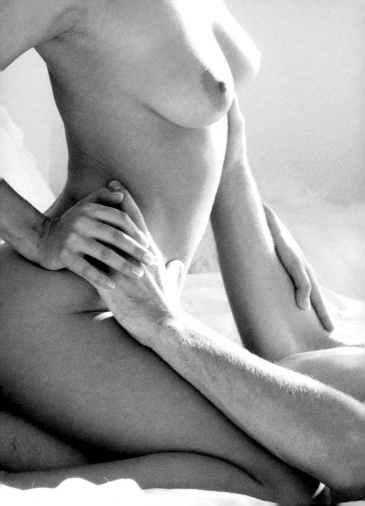

upper hands

In this classic woman-on-top position, the man lies on his back and the woman sits astride him, free to move in whatever way and at whatever speed she wants. There is lots of friction between the clitoris and the pubic bone which can be, quite literally, orgasmic. You can make the position warm and loving by gazing into each other's eyes and kissing. Or she can make it wild and raunchy by throwing her head back, pushing her breasts out and arching her spine. If she has a supple spine, she can place her hands by his feet and curve her spine back — and then gently gyrate her hips.

hand technique

He uses his fingers or thumb in circular movements or keeps his hand still against her clitoris, then lets her move backward and forward at her own pace.

skin-to-skin

This is a wonderful position for slow, soulful, intimate sex. The man lies on his back and the woman sits astride him. Once she's guided his penis into herself she can get into a lying position. Although you don't have much freedom to move, certain techniques can be highly stimulating. She can try resting her feet on top of his and push herself off against them; meanwhile he can help by guiding her body up and down. Or she can rest her feet on the floor, he can hold her, while she wiggles her hips from side to side. The higher up the woman's pelvis, the more clitoral stimulation she receives.

touch technique

He can use his fists, fingers and thumbs to apply deep, static pressure to the muscles of her buttocks, and then try gently spanking her buttocks too, if she enjoys this.

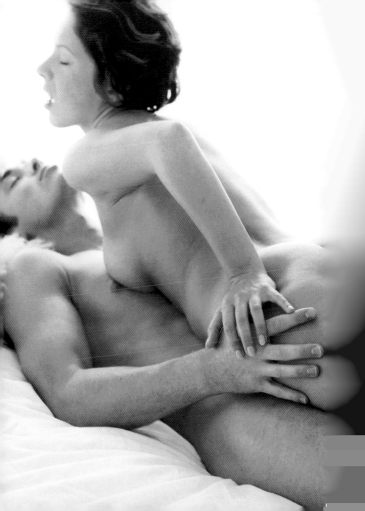

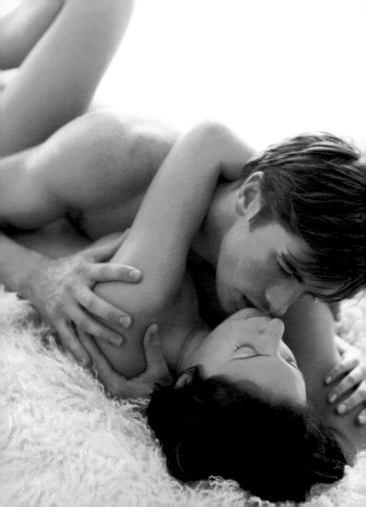

You can't get much closer to your lover than this — you're quite literally wrapped up in each other. Starting in either the missionary position, or a woman-on-top position, both the man and woman roll a little way on to their sides so his weight is not fully upon her. The scope for movement is quite limited but it's a great one for enjoying a long passionate kiss, and for holding each other tight and relishing the intimacy. Both can move by rocking against each other or one can thrust gently against the other. Or she can contract and relax her vaginal muscles around his penis.

touch technique

She presses her fingers into the muscles on either side of the top of his spine and then slowly and sensually slides them down the length of his back.

spoons position

This is comfortable, intimate and neither partner dominates. It facilitates unhurried, restful sex but with the intense sensations that deep penetration from behind can bring. After sex, you can stay in the Spoons Position and savour the relaxed closeness of your bodies.

She can experiment by having one leg straight and one leg bent. For deeper penetration, she can raise her knees so that they are closer to her body – the higher she raises them, the deeper he can penetrate. To give her better access to her clitoris, she can open her legs and hook her top leg over her lover.

touch technique

To add to the intimacy, she reaches behind his head and uses her nails and fingertips to softly caress the back of his neck and run her fingers through his hair.

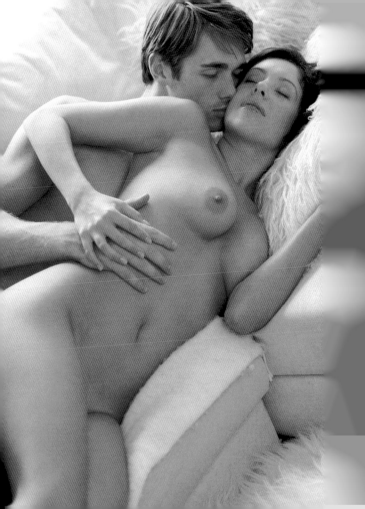

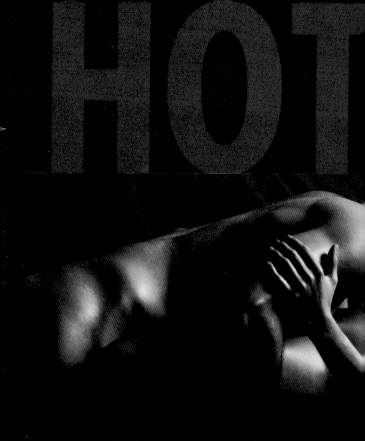

HOT

arouse • lick • stimulate • play • thrill • control

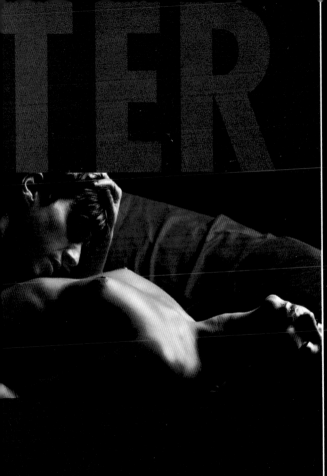

TER

HOTTER

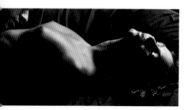 # HOT

Now that you're fully warmed-up, it's time to turn up the temperature a little. In part 1 – Hot – you learned to be more open about touch and more relaxed about caressing each other. Now you can begin to discover what really turns your lover on, free yourself of any inhibitions and delve much deeper into each other's pleasure zones.

While the hands are a hugely effective and erotic massage tool, it's time to experiment and

TER

discover how to use your genitals to give your lover a sensual hands-free caress that will take their arousal levels sky-high. As well as trying out some incredible G-spot techniques for a truly orgasmic experience, get slightly more adventurous with some *Kama Sutra* inspired lovemaking positions.

And for the times when you are alone, discover how to get hot all by yourself with some incredible caresses designed just for one.

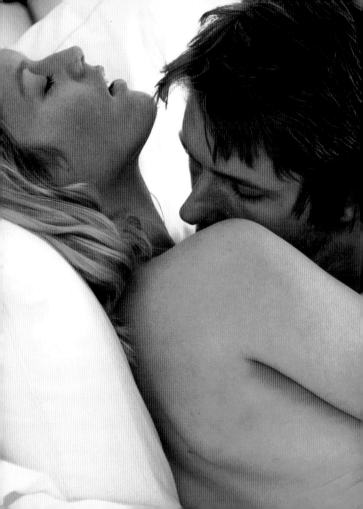

know each other

Some couples make love for years without knowing, for example, that her favourite way to receive oral sex is in the 69 position, or that he loves having his penis caressed slowly and gently.

asking questions

Ask your lover at what time of the day they feel most sexy. If, for example, your lover hates mornings, an erotic wake-up call won't work. Ask her where and how she likes to be touched on her clitoris and him where and how he likes to be touched on his penis. Masturbate to show each other the techniques you enjoy.

Ask what position your lover likes to be in while being touched. Some find it a turn-on to receive a genital massage while standing, whereas others like to be fully relaxed and lying down.

the erotic buttock

You can give your lover an array of sensations by touching their buttocks: a light "barely there" touch can bring about delicious shivers; a firm touch is deeply relaxing and penetrates to their core.

derrière delights

Lightly graze your fingernails over your lover's buttocks. Next, rub oil into them and massage the large muscles using deep strokes *(see page 21)*. Men might want to try gently nibbling their lover's buttocks. Women: try rubbing oil into your breasts, then slide and slither your way up your lover's legs and across his buttocks. And there is also spanking *(see page 132)*, too, for those who enjoy it.

Oil your fingers and gently stroke around the entrance to the anus. If your lover enjoys it, increase the pressure until you are massaging the opening. Avoid touching the vagina and anus in a single stroke.

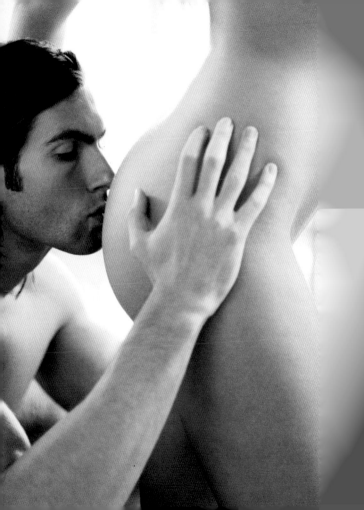

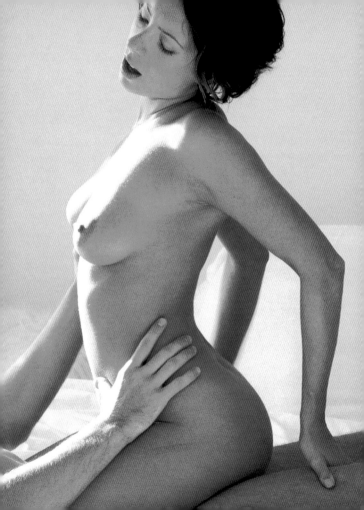

the voluptuous vagina

There's something incomparably sexy and erotic about being massaged by the vulva and vagina. It is such a powerful turn-on because the woman is completely in control.

massaging him

Support yourself on all fours above your lover so that your vulva is in contact with his belly and move your hips in slow, undulating movements so that your genitals caress him. Gradually move up his body, then slowly back down, moving your genitals against him.

Lower yourself on to his penis. Stay still for several seconds. Contract your vaginal muscles so that he feels tightly held, then relax them. Now contract your vaginal muscles, hold the contraction and move your vagina up his penis as though you were "milking" him. When you get to the tip, relax and sink back down.

the playful penis

Next time you make love, put aside the desire to ejaculate and, instead, imagine that your penis is a massage tool with which you are going to caress both the outside and inside of your lover.

massaging her

Make your erect penis slippery with lubricant. Holding the shaft in one hand, and supporting yourself on your other hand, rub the glans of your penis up and down the length of her vulva. Next, use the tip of your penis to massage her clitoris. Use a variety of different strokes: quick, light flicks backward and forward, and slow circles.

When your lover is really turned on, make tiny thrusting movements so that a small fraction of your penis enters her. Do this as many times as you — or she — can take it, and then penetrate her fully so that the entire length glides smoothly into her.

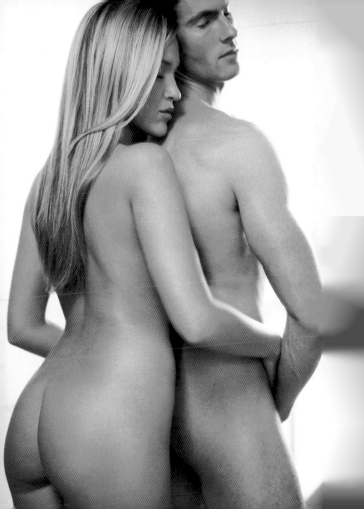

i love the way

and pleasure

you touch...

me all over

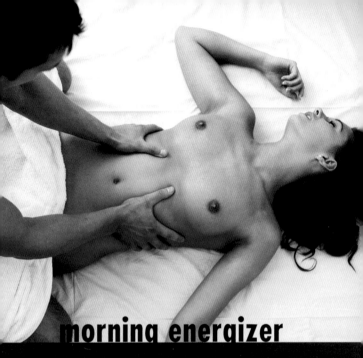

morning energizer

This erotic massage gradually awakens and arouses your lover. Begin by slipping your hands under the covers and sliding your palms in long, gentle movements along their body. Let your fingertips play at their breasts and genitals. Pour massage oil into your hands and kneel astride your

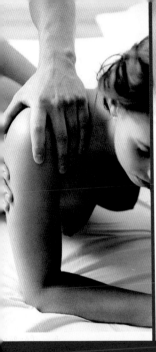
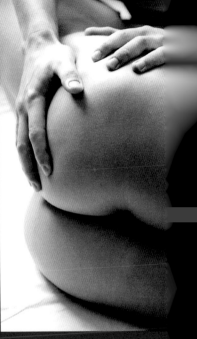

lover. Place your hands on their belly, then let them gently glide up to their chest and back down along their side. Ask your lover to roll over, then apply smooth, gliding strokes along the length of their back. Once your lover is fully awake, what happens next is entirely up to you.

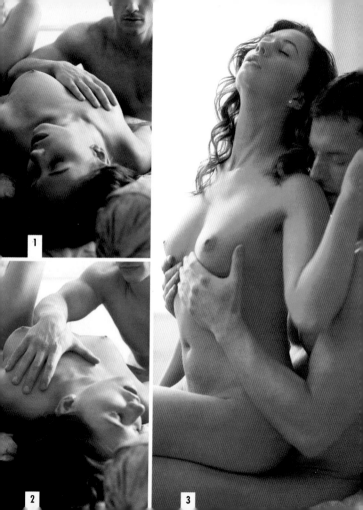

1

2

3

EROTIC BREAST MASSAGE

A sensual breast massage is a sure-fire way of taking many women to the peak of arousal – some orgasm from this alone. The secret is not to rush things.

1 Coat your hands in oil, sit or kneel and cup your lover's breasts in your hands. Stay in this position for a few moments so that you can both savour the sensations of touching and being touched.

2 Slowly and gently rotate her breasts, first clockwise, then anti-clockwise. Do this for a minute or two.

3 Place your hands below her breasts, resting them on the rib cage, and gently caress the sides of her breasts with your thumbs. Move your palms in a diagonal line from the side of her lower ribs to the opposite shoulder. Keep your palms flat and your fingers pointing to the shoulder they are moving toward. Alternate stroking each breast in this way. Then let your fingertips lightly and playfully brush her nipples.

UNDULATING OIL MASSAGE

This is an incredibly intimate and fun massage that will up the eroticism of your lovemaking. Make sure you use lots and lots of oil so that you get *really* messy!

get slippery

Protect your bed or the floor with towels or a PVC sheet. Rub each other's naked body with oil – aim to cover every surface. Lie on the floor and let your bodies slip and slide across each other. Don't think about what you're doing – just move in whichever way feels natural to you. Roll over, under and across each other; twist and slide.

Now take it turns to go on top and use your entire body as a massage tool. Experiment until you find the moves that feel good. You could start at your lover's feet and slide incredibly slowly up their body or lie across your lover and move back and forth.

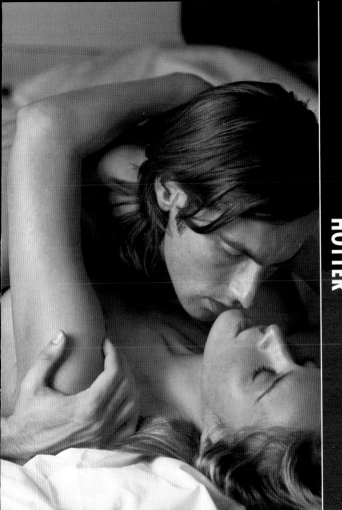

HOTTER

A MASSAGE FOR ONE

Get hot and experimental all by yourself with sensual self-touch. The idea is to explore your whole body at your own pace. Here are some ways to get started:

STEP 1 Lie on your back and take a few slow, deep breaths. Rest the palm of your hand on your belly and move it slowly in big, clockwise circles. Note any sensations in your hand as you touch yourself.

STEP 2 Let your knees drop to one side, but keep your shoulders flat on the floor so that you are lying in a twist. Use the hand nearest your raised buttock to firmly massage the large buttock muscle – make your middle fingers and forefingers as stiff as you can and walk them backward and forward across the muscle, pressing fairly hard.

STEP 3 Draw your knees up to your chest and hug them in your arms. Let your body become as heavy as possible – imagine it sinking into the floor. With your eyes closed, roll very slowly from side to side so that the floor massages the large muscles in your back. Roll your head from side to side too.

Return to lying flat on the floor. Using a featherlight touch, let your fingertips travel from your chest along the length of your neck and over your jawbone and chin so that they come to rest on your lips. Delicately trace the line of your lips.

Rest your middle three fingertips on the inner part of each eyebrow or slightly above. Draw your hands apart so that your fingers come to rest on your temples. Circle your fingers firmly on your temples several times and then repeat the stroke across your eyebrows. Finally, rake all your fingers through your hair.

End the massage by making long, sweeping strokes down the length of your whole body. Relax and let your hands glide all the way from your chest to your legs. Now move on to your genitals...

HOTTER

i want you to

There's nothing more sexually exciting
than discovering new pleasures together.
Being experimental with sex toys, trying
new lovemaking positions, touching each
other in new ways... If your lover seems shy
about being experimental, this in itself can
be a turn-on and helping them to overcome
any inhibitions can be rewarding and

all of my

uncover...

HOTTER

sexual desires

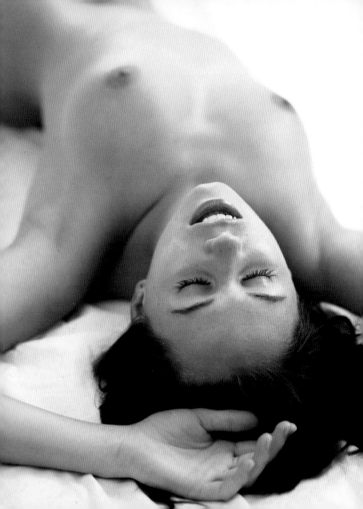

pleasure her g-spot

The G-spot is an area on the front wall of the vagina that swells during sexual arousal. The secret of a good G-spot massage is to use an exploratory approach and ensure your lover is highly aroused.

finger techniques

Gently slide your index and middle finger into her vagina and stroke the front wall of her vagina. When you feel a bump, ridge or protusion, bend your fingers into a "come here" gesture and gently stroke. Gradually increase the amount of pressure and ask your lover for feedback.

Some women liken the sensation to needing to urinate, but this feeling soon passes. Clitoral stroking or pressure on the lower abdomen can add to the pleasure, but take your cues from your lover.

pleasure his g-spot

The male G-spot is also called the P-spot as it is found on the prostate gland. You can't touch this gland, but you can massage it "remotely" through the perineum or through the wall of the rectum.

hidden delights

With your left hand on your lover's penis, use your right hand to massage the area between his scrotum and anus. Press quite deeply, using your fingertips and ask your lover to tell you when you hit the right spot. Once you've found this, move your fingers in deep circles. This spot is sometimes called the external prostate. Aim to move the muscles beneath the skin.

Now stimulate his G-spot through the wall of the rectum. Insert a well-lubricated finger into his anus, bend it in a "come here" gesture and massage the front wall of the rectum.

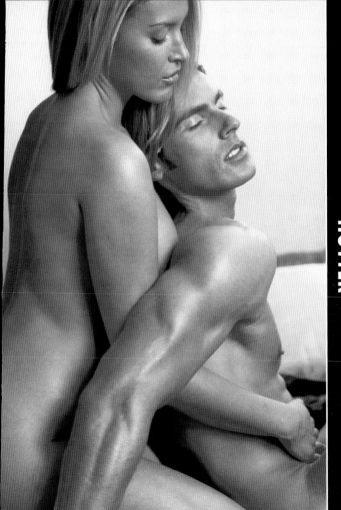

secret pleasure zones

The whole body can be a source of erotic pleasure, but there are
some hot spots, such as the inner and outer thighs, that feel
especially wonderful when caressed.

a voyage of discovery

Stroking the inner thighs feels incredibly sensual. Stand in front of
a mirror or sit up with your soles pressed together. Slowly and gently
slide your hands up the insides of your thighs. When you get to the
tops of your legs, move your fingertips along the crease of your
groin, round to your hips.

Now move your hands softly down the outsides of your
thighs. Continue this circular stroke, gradually reducing the pressure
until your hands are barely touching your skin. Now, if you wish,
stroke back up your inner thighs to your genitals.

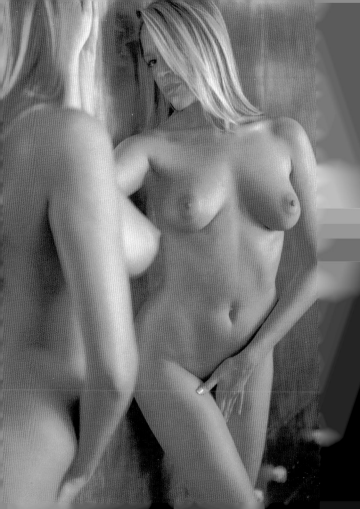

tie me up and

indulge in

ease me...

your fantasies

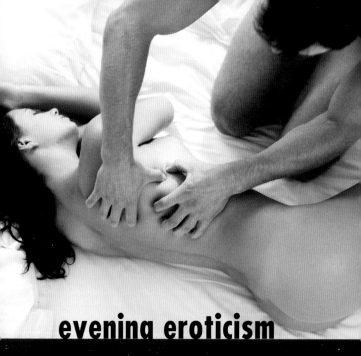

evening eroticism

Begin an evening of ecstatic pleasure with this erotic touch
technique guaranteed to have your lover begging for more.
Ask them to lie down, naked, on their side or front. Make your
hands into claw shapes and stroke their calves, thighs and
buttocks. Ask them whether they prefer a light or firm touch.

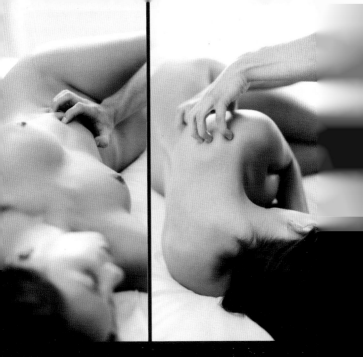

Move on to clawing their back, shoulders and arms. When your
lover is relaxed and their sensitivity heightened, ask them to
roll on to their back. Lightly claw the area around their belly,
and get tantalizingly closer to their genitals with each stroke.
Ask your lover to open their legs and claw your way down

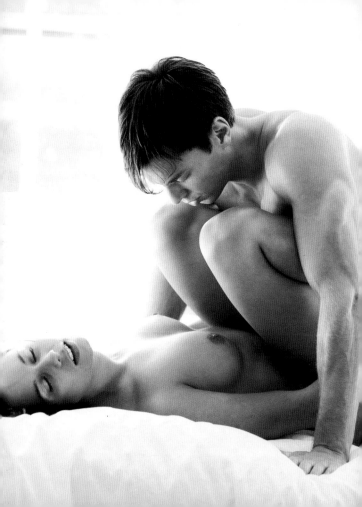

tightly pressed

The woman feels very deeply penetrated in this position because her knees are so tightly pressed to her chest. The greater the woman's arousal, the better able she is to accommodate the man – this is because, during the peak of arousal, the upper part of the vagina expands and the uterus lifts up. This is a great way to enjoy slow and sensual lovemaking as he kneels and gently thrusts in and out of her. The man will enjoy the dominance of being in this semi-upright and visually stimulating position, which gives him lots of opportunities for erotic touch and intimate eye contact.

touch technique

He stays perfectly still inside her and uses one fingertip to gently caress her face, neck and shoulders. He can also play with and massage her breasts and nipples.

the yawning position

The woman lies on her back and raises her legs so that they are at right angles to her body. The man guides his penis inside her in a kneeling position and she rests her legs along the front of his body. Her feet can rest over his shoulders or flat on his chest. This position offers a tantalizing combination of intimacy and distance — you can gaze into each other's eyes but you can't get close enough to kiss. If you both enjoy deep penetration, and she's flexible enough, she can bring her knees down to touch her shoulders. The penis penetrates deeply, so the man should thrust gently at first.

touch technique

She walks her index and middle fingers up the large muscles of his thighs and buttocks, pressing quite hard. When she gets to the waist, she walks them back again.

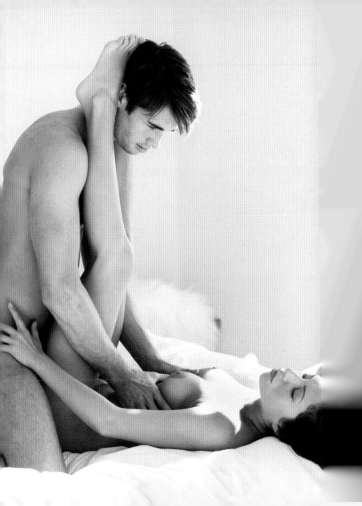

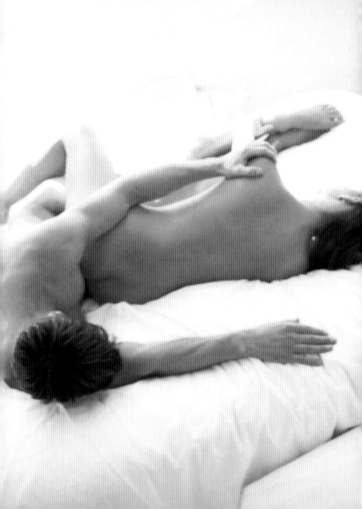

drawing the bow

If you enjoy having sex with him positioned behind, this is a great variation on doggie-style sex or spooning. You both lie on your side – him behind her – and she sandwiches his body between her legs. She leans forward to take hold of his calves or feet. He enters her and rests his hands on her shoulders. The man is limited in how freely he can thrust, but, instead of making vigorous movements, you can lie still together savouring the sensation of being joined. She can stimulate herself by touching her clitoris and stimulate him by contracting her vaginal muscles around his penis.

reach in below

She holds his feet in her hands and presses deeply into the soles with her fingers. She can also slide her fingers in and out of the spaces between his toes.

lap moves

This is great for passionate spur-of-the-moment sex. She's in control of most of the movement, so it's a great position for her to orgasm. She can slide up and down on his penis by standing and lowering herself. If she wants more control, she can put her feet on the seat of the chair and steady herself by clasping her hands behind his neck and then moving up and down. Alternatively, you can both rub oil into your thighs so that you slip and slide around on each other. Depending on his strength and her weight, he can move to a standing position with her legs clasped around his waist.

touch technique

He massages her with his mouth by flicking his tongue across her nipples, licking a line between her breasts and nuzzling the underside of them.

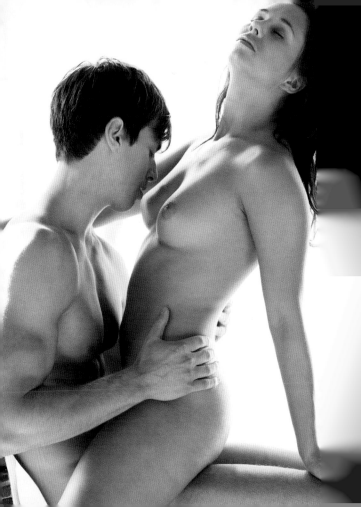

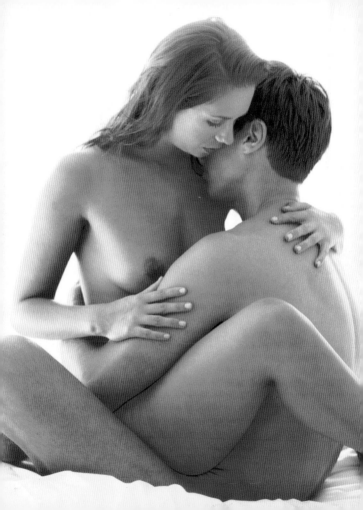

face to face

This is one of the best positions for feeling intimately connected with each other. It is stimulating enough to keep you aroused, but not so stimulating that orgasm is impossible to avoid. To get into position, he sits cross-legged and she sits astride him with her legs wrapped around him. You can move easily into a man-on-top or a woman-on-top position. Or, if you want to try something different, hold each other's hands and slowly lower yourselves backward so that you are lying down with your heads at opposite ends of the bed. Straighten your legs. Keep holding hands and pull and push against each other.

touch technique

She uses her thumb and forefinger to pinch, stroke and tweak his earlobe and can run her fingers gently through his hair. At the same time, she can kiss and nibble him softly on the lips.

RED

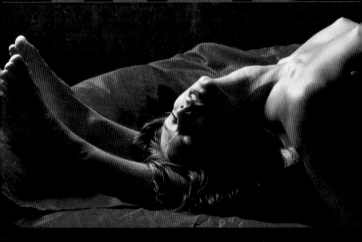

rude • raunchy • daring • erotic • experimental

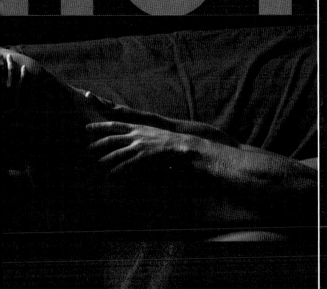

HOT

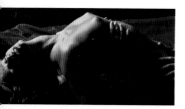

RED

Are you hot enough yet? You've touched, you've teased, and you've tantalized your lover. Now it's no-holds-barred as you get down and dirty with red-hot techniques that are guaranteed to have your lover screaming with pleasure.

The key to hotting things up is to become more experimental. You might want to begin by introducing some toys and tools to your lovemaking that will add a whole new range of sensual sensations and

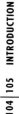

HOT

bring a new meaning to "playtime". And rather than using your hands to pleasure your lover, learn some tricks of the tongue that will leave them fully satisfied every time, including the Tantric take on erotic genital touch techniques.

Get more adventurous with some exotic and earth-moving positions that will banish bedroom boredom forever, and watch and learn from your lover as they touch themself and allow you a ringside seat.

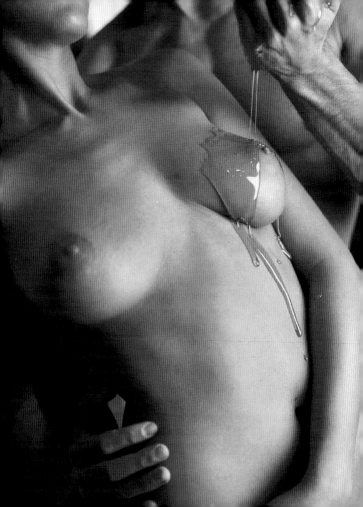

play together

Erotic touch is made all the more fun if you introduce some props. It is easy to use food and everyday objects in novel ways to excite and stimulate your lover.

Drizzle honey from the collarbone, down the breasts and on to the tummy so that it pools in the navel, before dripping down to the genitals. Remove the honey with your tongue... Move an ice cube in slow, circular movements around your lover's nipples. When they are rock hard, you can warm them up again using your lips and tongue.

The soft, fleeting touch of a feather can feel exquisite on the skin. Peacock feathers are exotic and arousing. A silk scarf can be used in the same way or used to blindfold your lover.

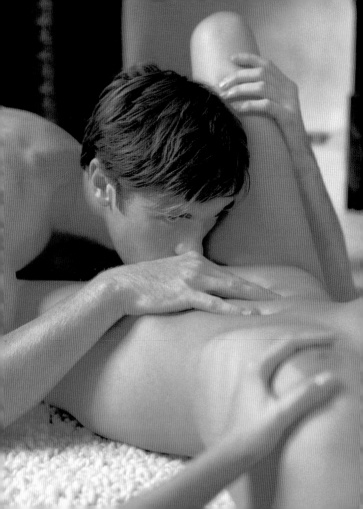

oral delights for her

Rather than relegating oral sex to a few minutes of pre-sex play, it is wonderful to give – and receive – mouth massage as a sexual gift entirely in its own right.

Tongue techniques

Use the tip of your tongue to draw circles clockwise, then anti-clockwise, around her clitoris. Aim to tantalize rather than stimulate her clitoris directly. Then lick the length of her vulva, pausing at her vaginal entrance to make firm swirling movements.

To stimulate her clitoris directly, put your lips around the tip and suck. Then, still sucking, move the flat part or the tip of your tongue in slow, firm circles on or around her clitoris. Flick your tongue fast across her clitoris too. As her arousal builds, increase the speed of your tongue strokes and maintain a regular rhythm.

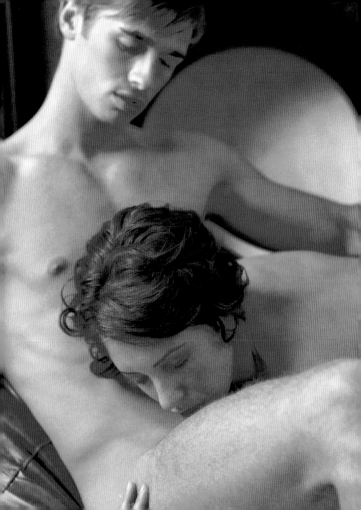

oral delights for him

The mouth is perfect for massage: it is warm and soft, the tongue is capable of delivering a multitude of sensations… and it comes ready-lubricated.

the ultimate pleasure

When he has a solid erection, hold the tip of his penis against his belly and lick the length of the underside by moving your head from side to side. Then move your tongue to his frenulum and use the pointed tip of your tongue to rapidly flick this area.

Just below your lips, encircle his penis with your thumb and forefinger. The combination of your soft lips and harder hand will be highly stimulating for him. Move both "rings" simultaneously up and down. Now keep your mouth going up and down while your thumb and forefinger twist and stroke the middle of his shaft.

be at one with

discover the

each other...

erotic pleasure, you can also give and receive
erotic energy. As you hold your hands above
your lover's skin you will begin to feel the
pulse and tingle of energy flowing through
your fingertips. You can use this to heal your
lover, free them of tension and take them to
a new plane of sensual awareness. Try the
massage on the following pages.

oy of Tantra

tantric touch for her

The aim of this massage is to reduce muscle tension in and around your lover's vagina. You will be massaging away tension that may have been stored there for many years.

rings of tissue

Imagine your lover's vagina consists of several rings or bands of tissue, one on top of the other. The first ring is just inside the entrance to her vagina; the last is high up in her vagina by the cervix. You are slowly and firmly going to massage each ring.

Tantric massage can also be effective on the G-spot (see page 83), which, if massaged for a prolonged period, can be an intense experience for women. Tension due to unsatisfying or frustrating sexual experiences can get lodged there and massage can bring a profound sense of "letting go", and intense sexual pleasure.

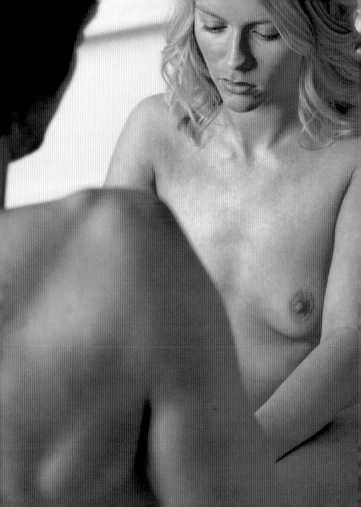

tantric touch for him

This relaxes and loosens the muscles around the penis and the scrotum. It increases penile sensitivity and enhances sexual sensations. Be guided by your lover throughout.

perineal massage

Lubricate your hands well and apply gradual circular pressure along the junction between your lover's thigh and perineum (the area between the anus and scrotum). Work your way down this junction. If you sense tension in a particular area, stop and work on it. Next, work on the junction between the opposite thigh and perineum.

Now massage the perineum, pressing your fingertips in circular movements. Your aim is to release tension in the muscles in this area. Next, massage the muscles at the base of the penis.

Genital massage feels like an especially indulgent treat because all of her erotic hot spots receive prolonged, slow and direct attention.

STEP 1 Generously lubricate your palms with massage oil and then stroke your lover's vulva from the back to the front, palm over palm so that your hands don't break contact with her. Make your strokes long, slow and firm and let them finish on her pubic mound. For hygiene reasons, don't include her anus. Repeat these strokes for a couple of minutes.

STEP 2 Instead of using your palm to stroke her vulva, use your fingertip. Let it glide along the right side of her vulva up over her clitoral hood and then back down the left side. Do this incredibly slowly and ask her if she'd like you to press harder. Keep moving your fingertip in this U shape for two or three minutes. Avoid touching her clitoris or clitoral hood – make her wait...

STEP 3 Use the pads of your index and middle fingers to press the area on your lover's pubic mound immediately above her clitoral hood. Slowly move your fingers in circles, getting closer and closer to her clitoris. Before you reach her clitoris, take your fingers away and replace them with just one fingertip. Use this to draw slow, clockwise circles around her clitoral hood. Keep doing this for a few minutes — vary the speed and pressure in response to any feedback she gives you. Finally, move your finger or fingers in circles directly on her clitoris or clitoral hood.

STEP 4 Put one or more well-lubricated fingers inside your lover's vagina (ask her what feels comfortable), and gently slide them in and out, exploring and caressing her vaginal walls.

STEP 5 Now experiment with some different finger movements, and try inserting your finger into her vagina and stimulating her clitoris at the same time.

Over time the same predictable touch can lose its power. This is why a new set of strokes for his penis that he might not use himself can be super-erotic.

STEP 1 Cover your lover's penis and scrotum — fingers spread apart and facing his feet — and use the other hand to pour oil over the back of the first hand. The oil will drip between your fingers and lubricate his genitals, making the massage easier for you and more pleasurable for him. Next, use your hands to stroke his scrotum and penis in long, smooth movements, one hand after the other. These strokes should gently pull his scrotum and penis in the direction of his head.

STEP 2 Grasp his penis with your hand and gently squeeze it inside your fist. Use both hands if necessary, one fist on top of the other. Do this pumping action in a rhythmic fashion, using different amounts of pressure for variety. This stroke mimics the way you might use your pelvic floor muscles to squeeze his penis during sex.

The F-spot refers to the frenulum — the fold of skin on the underside of the penis. This is a particularly sensitive spot. Use one hand to hold the bottom of the shaft, and the thumb of the other hand to make small circular movements on the frenulum.

Interlock your fingers and wrap your hands around your lover's penis. The heels of your hands should meet on the underside of his penis. His shaft should now be tightly enclosed in the tube made by your hands. Make your thumbs point upward so that the pads of your thumbs rest on his frenulum. Using a firm grip, move the tube of your hands up and down on his penis.

This massage stroke is sometimes called the "juicer". It resembles the way you might juice a lemon by twisting it back and forth on a lemon squeezer. Use one hand to draw his foreskin down his shaft. Use the fingers of your other hand to grip just below the glans. Move his hand in a twisting, up-and-down movement.

i trust you,

A blindfold is a fantastic tool to include in your erotic toy box. Using one may help to bring you closer to your lover because it only works if there is total trust between you.

Although your lover can get a buzz from watching what you are doing, depriving them of sight can offer a rich and highly erotic experience. Without sight your lover

i'll do al

surrender...

becomes much more aware of and sensitized to touch. Blindfolding them also sends the message that you are in control — and this, in itself, can be an amazing turn-on — for both of you. And a lover who can't see will be far more open to suggestion, so you can plant a whole array of wonderfully erotic images or fantasies in their mind!

hat you say

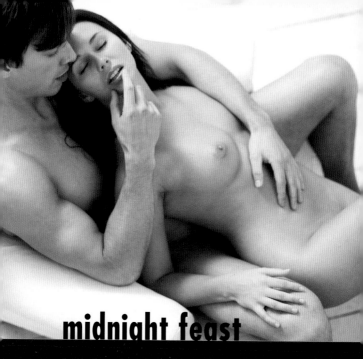

midnight feast

In this feast the only food you will "eat" is your lover. Start by running your index finger lightly around their lips. Pause to push your fingertip suggestively into their mouth. Softly place your lips against your lover's and use the tip of your tongue to trace the outline of their lips. Use your lips to gently enclose and

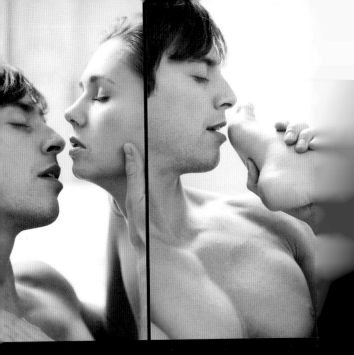

nuzzle the lower lip. Move down for the main course. Start with a genital fingertip massage, using the tip of your index finger to trace lines along the vulva or penis and then do the same with your tongue. For dessert, sensually suck your lover's toes. Now the "meal" is over, play some after-dinner games...

self-pleasure for her

Make sure your privacy is guaranteed and that you have plenty of time. Rather than rushing to reach orgasm, slowly explore your genitals and be experimental.

genital caress

Let your hands play on your skin: skim the surface of your breasts with your fingertips, or gently drag your nails across your belly. Now get a mirror, open your legs and look at and admire your genitals. Gently touch different places and imagine that you are trying to rate each place for sensitivity.

If you usually masturbate with one or two fingers, use three or four – or use your palm. Whatever you do usually, try something different. Instead of using your fingers, squeeze your thighs together or touch yourself with a prop, such as a feather.

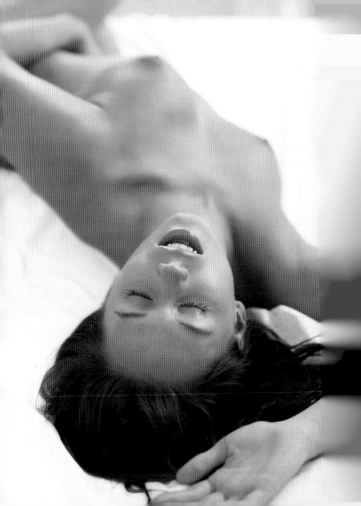

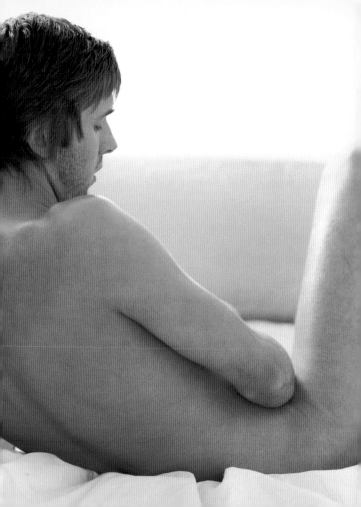

self-pleasure for him

Instead of masturbating quickly, using the strokes you always use, take time to treat yourself to a languorous and sensual experience. Let your body move in whatever way comes naturally.

more than masturbation

Be experimental by trying different touch techniques. For example, place your palms on either side of the shaft of your penis and rub them backward and forward (as if you were rubbing sticks together to make fire). From this stroke you can interlock your fingers and use both hands to stroke your penis up and down.

Rather than lying on your back, try squatting or kneeling with the heel of one foot pressed against your perineum. If you feel close to coming, decrease the speed or the pressure or use your hands to massage your thigh and belly instead of your penis.

watching each other

It can be a great turn-on to watch your lover give themself an erotic massage and it will give you a fabulous insight into what kind of touch they most enjoy.

putting on a show

Touch your body in whatever way comes naturally to you. You can start by stroking your arms or legs to get into a relaxed mood or you can stimulate your genitals straight away — you're in charge. If you feel self-conscious, close your eyes and imagine you are alone.

If you are the one who is watching, you are not allowed to touch. Sit close by so that your lover can sense your arousal, and talk dirty as they caress themselves. Describe how much you're turned on, tell them where and how you want them to touch and — in detail — what you plan to do to them later...

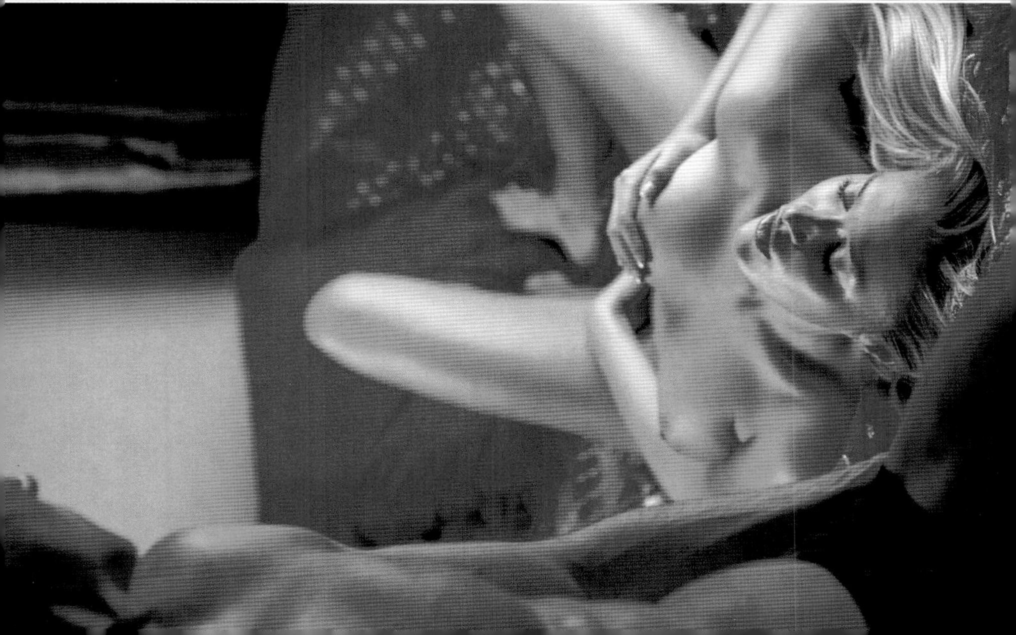

i've been very

and need

naughty...

to be spanked

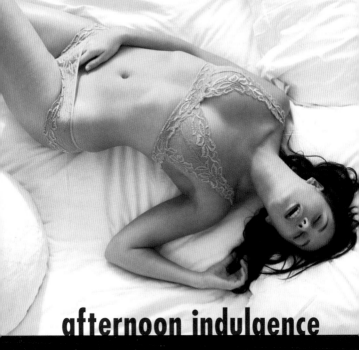

afternoon indulgence

Sensual self-pleasure can be enjoyed at any time. Make sure you won't be disturbed and when you feel completely relaxed, stroke your body. Allow your hands to intuitively change the amount of pressure they apply on different parts of the body. Once you are immersed in this pleasure

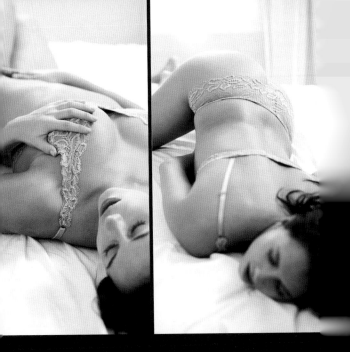

rest your hand on your genitals and imagine drawing up erotic energy into your body with each breath. Visualize this energy as red; imagine it permeating your whole body. Enjoy the sensuality of this for as long as you like and bring yourself to orgasm if and when you feel ready.

rear straddle

This position is loved by both men and women for its sheer sexiness. He lies on his back and she simply sits astride him with her back to him. The woman is very much in control both in terms of depth of penetration and movement. She can grind, thrust, circle her hips or move up and down on his penis. Alternatively, she can sit still and just contract her vaginal muscles around his penis. He is forced into the eroticism of submission because he can't move very much. As you're facing away from each other, this becomes a great position for abandoning yourself to a favourite erotic fantasy.

touch technique

He presses his fingers into the top of her back and slides them down either side of her spine in a single stroke. For an electrifying effect he should do this when she's about to climax.

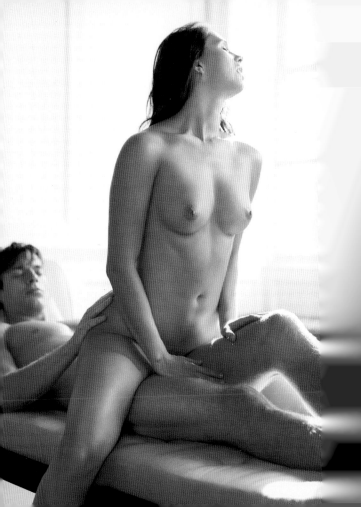

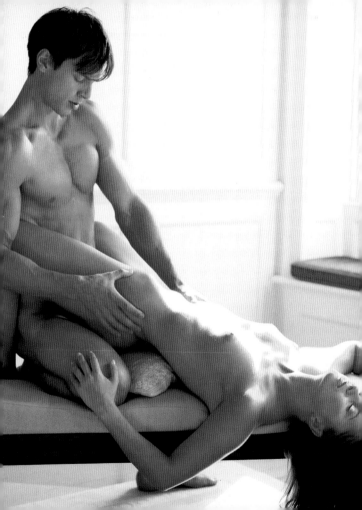

wide open

She lies on her back with a cushion beneath her bottom and he kneels in between her legs and enters her. The cushion raises her pelvis, which makes her vagina more accessible and facilitates deeper penetration. This is an "equal" position in that the man and woman can take it in turns to lead. He can thrust and move from side to side, while she can raise her pelvis and move her hips in circular or undulating movements. Because of the angle of this position, and the fact that she can control the thrusting, there is a good chance of her having a clitoral orgasm.

touch technique

She can really turn him on by touching herself... she can stroke her body, caress her breasts, play with her nipples and rub her clitoris. This will be a wonderful visual delight for him.

knees and elbows

While she supports herself on her knees and elbows, he penetrates her from behind. Lots of couples love the raw animalism of this position and the freedom of movement it offers. He can also penetrate her quite deeply. To achieve maximum penetration, she should push up her bottom as high as possible. He can ramp up the sexual tension by varying the rhythm and depth of his thrusts. For example, he could mix shallow strokes that just penetrate her vaginal entrance with deep strokes that stimulate her G-spot *(see page 83)*. Or he could alternate thrusting with wiggling his hips.

touch technique

He should make the most of having access to her buttocks by using the tips of his fingers to caress her. If she prefers a firmer touch, he can press his knuckles into her buttocks and twist firmly.

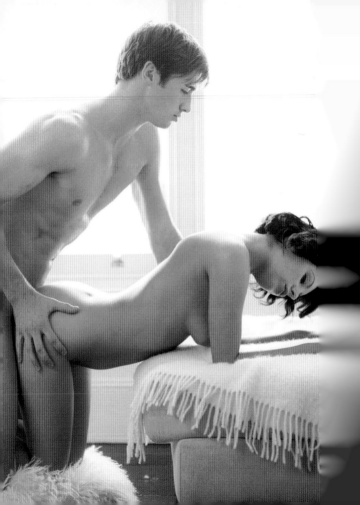

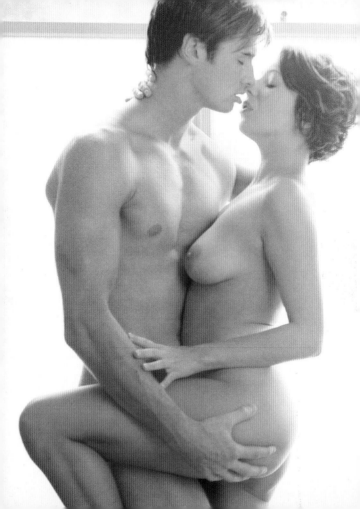

get up close

This is a great position for spontaneous sex. She simply puts her arms around his neck and wraps one leg around his waist. He will probably need to bend his knees a little to penetrate her. If he is taller, she can help by wearing high heels, standing on tiptoe, raising her leg high on his body, or standing on a raised surface such as a step. Alternatively, he can bend into a deep squat, or pick her up so that both her legs are around his waist. There isn't a lot of freedom of movement in this position, but the slow, careful movements of his penis can make up for this in eroticism.

She can use her lips and tongue to nuzzle, lick and kiss the sensitive spots along the sides of his neck and along the line of his jaw, and her hands to caress his face and hair.

index

Author's acknowledgments
Thanks to Grace Cheetham,
Manisha Patel, Jantje Doughty
and Dawn Bates at Duncan
Baird Publishers.